I0413619

REBOOT YOUR LIFE TODAY
The Easy Start Guide To Making Health Changes That Stick

CHERYL GIPSON

DEDICATION

This book is dedicated to my mom, Mildred C. Gipson who first taught me the importance of health.

CONTENTS

ACKNOWLEDGMENTS

I could not have written this book without my family who provided me daily support; thank you Mom, Celia (Tammy) Hudson, Karen Jenkins and Louis Gipson. All of those encouraging conversations, prayers, and belief fueled me to keep going and get it done.

Special thanks goes to Jenai Gatlin, my writing coach and friend who was with me every step of the way. I truly could not have completed this project without her (and her husband Dwayne, for letting her spend all that time helping me).

I also need to thank my very close friends who all told me I could do it when this book was just a dream–you all know who you are.

INTRODUCTION

"So many people spend their health gaining wealth, and then have to spend their wealth to regain their health."

A.J. Materi

The goal of this book is to bring awareness that gaining better health, even optimal health, is easy and attainable to the average person whether they are parents, single or married, working or retired.

I am not providing medical advice in any way, but the information contained in this book was helpful to me on my journey to better health and I'd like to share what I learned with you.

When I was struggling with health concerns and started to seek more natural ways to improve my conditions, it became clear that I was the only one responsible for improving my health. The government and food manufacturers have their own agendas that didn't line up with my expectations. Politics even plays a major role in health, as we'll discuss in later chapters.

Although there is a lot of information available on disease prevention, health, and wellness, the solution for most of us is simple: better nutrition.

Like many people, I was always managing a full schedule. Between my career that included a lot of traveling and my personal life, I was very busy and didn't always pay attention to my health. I guess I thought I'd always have good health—like the saying by Denis Waitley:

"Time and **health** are two precious assets that we don't recognize and appreciate until they have been depleted."

When faced with my health challenges, I took action and used what I learned to turn my health around, and so can you. My process was not to make drastic, immediate changes that wouldn't stick, but rather to approach the changes for the long term; to make healthier choices. I had specific goals around weight loss and improved health markers, but I wanted to ensure that I set a foundation for habits I could keep for a lifetime.

Once I started making better choices to improve my health, some of the benefits were immediately noticeable. Weeks into my process, friends and colleagues began asking me about the noticeable changes in my hair, skin, energy level and weigh loss. Since I wasn't on a formal eating or exercise plan, I was able to share my own tips and new habits that created the transformation in me.

Depending on life's circumstances I would give myself flexibility to adjust my actions and eating habits, while still keeping my overall health goals in mind. For example, if I was traveling, I wouldn't focus on following a strict eating regimen like eating six small meals; instead I would simply make healthier food choices whenever I got a meal. I wouldn't be concerned with eating gluten-free if the only option was a boxed lunch with a sandwich during an all-day meeting.

Having this flexibility made it easier to focus on my overall health goals instead of following a strict diet. Managing my health when faced with the challenges, demands and stresses of life is how *Reboot Your Life Today – The Easy Start Guide to Making Health Changes that Stick* was born. There are many components to eating well and making healthy choices, but as we go about our busy lives, we can't let our lifestyle derail our health goals.

Getting better nutrition for you and your family can be easy if you follow the steps in this book. I'll show you simple ways to make healthier choices that still let you live your normal life.

Before we get to the easy ways to reboot your life, we'll take a look at health in America, food manufacturing and the key factors that play a role in achieving better health and ultimately a longer and happier life. This background will give you the information you need to make informed choices, and implement permanent, positive changes for you and your family.

1
THE HEALTH CRISIS

"Don't Dig Your Grave with Your Own Knife and Fork."

English Proverb

America's Health Crisis

The United States of America, affectionately known as the Land of Opportunity, boasts the most millionaires in the world, the world's largest economy, and unfortunately, the highest percentage of obese people.

We lead the world in innovation, but finish last in health.

According to the Centers for Disease Control, the Women's Cancer Research Fund, United States Department of Health and Human Services and The American Cancer Society; the current statistics predict a bleak outlook for Americans:

- 1 in 3 people live with some form of cardio-vascular disease.
- 1 in 3 women will develop cancer.
- 1 in 2 men will develop cancer.
- 1 in 3 people will develop diabetes by 2050.

Why are the statistics so depressing if we as Americans are spending over \$2.6 trillion dollars a year on healthcare?

We spend more money on healthcare than any other country on earth, yet the health of Americans continues to deteriorate. There are many reasons for this, including poverty, lack of access to fresh foods, inadequate medical care, misinformation, greed, politics, culture and tradition. We'll look in more detail at a few of these reasons in later chapters, but understanding there is a very real national crisis is key to getting ready to make the lasting changes necessary to get you and your family healthier.

Food manufacturers, farmers and in some cases, the government, are making it harder and harder to determine which foods are healthy and which foods are harmful. Currently, nutrition labels do not fully disclose the nutritional value or harm of food products. General rule: if a food requires a label, proceed with caution! You practically need a degree in chemistry to understand what's in some of the processed foods we consume. Lobbyists, backed by the food industry, are continuing to win on limiting how much information has to be disclosed to the consumer on packaged foods. One of my goals is to make you aware of how modern food is manufactured and processed so you will be equipped to make better food choices to improve your health.

Kids in Crisis

Since the 1970s, obesity in children has more than doubled and children are getting chronic diseases at younger and younger ages. The health statistics regarding our children are very troubling:

- Many children will develop hardening of the arteries before they reach their teens.
- 1 in 3 children is obese.
- 1 in 3 children will develop diabetes in their lifetime.
- More than 25% of American children take prescription medication.
- Children as young as 8 years old are now being treated with cholesterol-lowering statin drugs.

Many factors contribute to the obesity and poor health of American children, including environment (inside and outside), genetics, culture, diet and a sedentary lifestyle. Heavy marketing of unhealthy foods to our children is not helping; and is certainly part of the problem. The food industry spends over $1.6 billion annually advertising mostly unhealthy, nutrient-void food to our children.

Because most adults aren't practicing good nutrition, they pass their unhealthy eating habits on to their kids. The best health teacher for children is seeing their parents eat healthy.

Forcing children to eat their vegetables, when you don't, is not setting a good example. As you plan your weekly meals, add your favorite fruits and vegetables, so your children will see that you are making good food choices. Fast food is no longer the only convenient meal on the market these days. More than ever before, our grocery stores are now full of healthy pre-packaged snacks and on-the-go meals.

Lack of exercise is also contributing to our children's health crisis. Today's kids' lifestyles are just as busy as their parents'. While their schedules are filled with extracurricular activities, they may not be getting any exercise at all, unless some of their activities are sports related. If your family's weekdays are busy with careers, commuting and homework; plan family outdoor activities for the weekend, even if you have to forgo some social events. Children are going to remember the fun times with their family more than attending a non-family event.

Tip: If you have children, commit to not purchasing as many processed foods like cookies, chips and sugary cereals. Plan to add fruits and vegetables to create healthier meals.

Tip: Seek out convenient meals in the grocery store instead of fast food restaurants.

Tip: Turn kids' computer gaming time into family time with interactive games that force you to move, like dancing or sporting games.

My Health Crisis

I was a pretty healthy person as a young adult until I suffered a bad case of pneumonia. I recall that after my father died, while in a state of grief, I developed a sinus infection which quickly turned into bronchitis. It was so bad that several rounds of antibiotics didn't improve my condition and I landed in the hospital for a full week with pneumonia.

I didn't experience any other major health problems, other than the occasional respiratory flare ups, but I did struggle with yo-yo dieting. Because of my attempts to either lose weight or keep it off, and my fascination with improving my health, I was always reading, researching, dieting, and cleansing. I've had many successes, but those pounds always seemed to come back. I could never find a plan that I could do for a lifetime; there was always traveling, business dinners or another excuse that wouldn't allow me to stick to a diet plan.

Several years ago, I started noticing small but nagging ailments around the time I started a more stressful job. My energy level was low, my skin was discolored, and my hair was dull and breaking.

As the months wore on, I also started having digestive and stomach issues as well as headaches and insomnia. Since some of my symptoms pointed to a possible thyroid disorder, I got testing done, but the results did not show anything abnormal. This was the beginning of my quest to find solutions to my health issues.

I began chiropractic care and eventually saw some improvements. The symptoms would come back from time to time, but the sleep issues were outweighing all the others. When I initially sought medical treatment, the doctors recommended sleep aids, which I refused because I'd read about all the horrible side effects like sleep walking, night eating and addiction.

One day, I was discussing my insomnia with my mother and she told me to drink a cup of chamomile tea. I laughed and said, "That's not going to help me—I can fall asleep, I just can't stay asleep!"

A few weeks later, I was at an office visit with a new doctor and I shared my concerns with her and she suggested—of all things—chamomile tea. The tea did help on many occasions, but as time went on, all my symptoms, including insomnia increased as my stress level increased. From time to time, I would start eating healthy, and see some improvements, but something would always seem to interfere with me sticking to the healthy eating habit.

The final straw came when I began coughing up phlegm every morning. I wasn't sure exactly what was wrong, but I knew the solution was not pharmaceutical medicine. At this point, I knew my issues were more than stress related so I sought treatment from a natural doctor and other health professionals at an integrated medical practice. Although the treatment was very expensive, I knew for sure that traditional medicine was not what I needed. Based on my research, I suspected that I was allergic to something that was causing my body to react abnormally.

After a battery of tests, I was 'prescribed' almost 20 supplements and told to follow gluten-free and diary-free diets for one month. I was completely shocked at the number of supplements, but luckily it was only for a short period of time because I was not used to taking so many pills.

One of the tests was an allergy test which revealed that I had gluten intolerance and a cow's milk allergy which I'd never had before. Those and a few other new allergies were affecting my digestion, exacerbating my respiratory issues, and causing low energy level and skin problems. Also, my adrenals glands were not functioning properly due to the stress.

After this diagnosis, I had to make some serious changes to my food intake and lifestyle. Essentially, I needed to reduce stress and change my eating habits for life. Having to follow such a drastic eating plan for life was very daunting, even though I knew it would improve my health. How was I ever going to give up bread, pasta, cheese and ice cream for life? I loved those foods!

Still, I was willing to try the dietary changes if it meant feeling better, and I did feel a noticeable improvement after the first month of my new diet. Encouraged, I decided to continue the gluten- and diary-free diet for many additional months.

My skin improved, my energy level increased, and I lost some weight. As I began to feel better, I slowly started adding unhealthy foods back into my diet. About a year after my initial dietary changes, I gained some of the weight back and would from time to time experience the old symptoms. In short, I didn't maintain the appropriate lifestyle changes to stay healthy.

Eventually, after being sick and tired of being sick and tired and not feeling my best, I decided to make the changes for life. As I mentioned previously, I would choose healthy options to focus on and make those a habit. After a few months, when those changes became second nature, I'd work on something else and my health started to change in a more positive direction. The pounds haven't come off quickly, but they are staying off this time, my skin is glowing, my energy level is constant and I just *feel* healthier.

Reversing the Health Crisis Starts with You

Among all the bad news and scary statistics, there is some good news. Americans have access to the most advanced medical technologies; have more money to spend on getting healthy, and new health laws allow more people to have insurance coverage.

The cheapest and easiest way for Americans to change the current health crisis is to make our individual health a priority and choose to make better lifestyle and nutrition choices. Nearly all of the modern day diseases can be attributed to the decline in the quality of our foods and poor nutrition. Many studies have proven that good nutrition can vastly improve your health and prevent diseases.

This book is not a quick fix answer, but will arm you with tips and easy action items that will work with your busy lifestyle.

The best news of all is you already have everything it takes to get healthier. You are aware of the need to improve, and after reading this book, you'll have even more resources to reach your health goals.

2
DON'T LET FOOD BE YOUR POISON

"The food you eat can be either the safest and most powerful form of medicine or the slowest form of poison."

Ann Wigmore

What Bad Nutrition Has Done To Us

Chronic Disease

Medical experts say that bad nutrition is a leading cause of chronic disease and death in America. Chronic disease is best described as a long-lasting condition that is manageable but not curable. These conditions include diabetes, arthritis, coronary heart disease, cancer and stroke. Dr. William Sears, a world renowned pediatrician, states that 75% of all chronic disease is preventable.

The problem is that most people's current eating habits are not preventing disease, but leading them straight down the path to disease and other degenerative health conditions.

The Centers for Disease Control and Prevention states that there are **four modifiable health risk behaviors** that may lead to chronic disease and are responsible for much of the illness, suffering, and early death related to those chronic diseases:

1) Lack of physical activity
2) Poor nutrition
3) Tobacco use
4) Excessive alcohol consumption

Combined, chronic diseases have reached an epidemic scale and will account for more than 50 million deaths and cost the global economy $47 trillion by 2030, according to Dr. Mark Hyman, an acclaimed medical author and international expert in identifying the cause of chronic diseases.

Obesity

In the United States, 78.4 million people over the age of 20 are obese. Obesity occurs in an individual when his or her body weight is 20% or more above a normal body weight. The body mass index (BMI), a calculation of height and weight is the most common measure of obesity. If a person has a BMI of 30% or more, they are obese. Obesity is an epidemic that's been a national discussion for several decades, yet the number of obese people keep increasing.

The most common causes of obesity are consuming too many calories and not exercising enough to burn them off. There are other factors such as heredity, gender, illness, medication and physiological issues, but in most cases, it's due to overeating and under-exercising.

Obesity leads to a higher risk for high blood pressure and cholesterol, coronary artery disease, gallstones, diabetes, stroke, sleep apnea, and other conditions.

TIP: You can measure your BMI online on the Reboot Your Life Books website: http://www.rebootyourlifebooks.com/

Inflammation

Inflammation is your body's response to allergens, foods, or other things that cause irritation; essentially, your body is going into protection mode. Sometimes inflammation is self-protecting and positive, such as swelling which will help the body heal itself. Most of the time however, inflammation caused by food is negative and can have devastating and uncomfortable results for our bodies, creating joint pain, bloating, fatigue and other issues.

Chronic inflammation is a long term condition that if left unchecked can cause conditions like rheumatoid arthritis, and experts believe it can even lead to heart disease, obesity and cancer. Food plays a major role in aggravating or helping alleviate inflammation. Sugar, fatty foods, and foods you may be allergic to, increase inflammation.

On the flip side, eating an anti-inflammatory diet can reduce inflammation. Foods on this diet include salmon, dark leafy greens, nuts, soy, peppers, tomatoes, beets, ginger and turmeric, garlic, onions, olive oils, grass fed beef, unrefined cocoa, and broccoli.

TIP: An elimination diet can help you identify foods that may cause you irritation. Foods to be avoided: sugar, gluten, dairy, peanuts and eggs are very common irritants. See the Allergens section in Chapter 3 for more information on this this type of diet.

What's Going Wrong

The Food Pyramid
In June 2011, the U.S. Department of Agriculture (USDA), along with the Department of Health and Human Services (DHHS) replaced the Food Pyramid with the MyPlate campaign, which recommends that half the food on our plate be fruits and vegetables.

Whatever happened to that Food Pyramid that pushed all those carbohydrates? Those recommendations have gone by the wayside, as Americans are larger than ever, and as we've consumed more and more processed foods. Is that old guideline partially responsible for the fattening of America? Could processed foods be toxic to our bodies? We'll explore the answer to those questions in the next few sections.

Modern Day Food Processing/Corporate Farmers

Today's food manufacturing process takes most of the nutrients out of the original food – to the point that it's almost unrecognizable. For instance, wheat and corn are taken through such a rigorous process to create cereal; most of the nutrients are almost non-existent. According to Food Matters website:

> When we put cereals through an extruder, it alters the structure of the proteins. Zeins, which comprise the majority of proteins in corn, are located in spherical organelles called protein bodies. The scientific literature does contain one study on extruded grains, which investigated changes in protein body, shape and release of encapsulated alpha-zeins as a result of the extrusion processing. Researchers found that during extrusion, the protein bodies are completely disrupted and the alpha-zeins dispersed. The results suggest that the zeins in cornflakes are not confined to rigid protein bodies but can interact with each other and other components of the system, forming new compounds that are foreign to the human body. The extrusion process breaks down the organelles and disperses the proteins, which then become toxic. When the proteins are disrupted in this way, it can adversely affect the nervous system, as indicated by the cornflake experiment.

The food industry spends over $40 million in lobbying efforts each year to persuade our elected officials to allow them to cut corners by including harmful chemicals in their food processing and other industrialized agricultural techniques that allow them to save money and increase their bottom line at the expense of the nation's overall health.

Beware of GMOs

Genetically modified organisms (GMOs) are foods or animals that have been changed to the point that the new organism is completely different from the original. According to the Non-GMO Project, GMOs are defined as:

> Plants (sometimes animals) created through a gene splicing technique that is also referred to as genetic engineering, or GE. This biotechnical process creates unnatural combinations of genes that change the original structure of the plant. Many times, these GMOs are detrimental to us, especially when they are commercially processed.

GMOs are less nutritious and can cause many health risks to the human body including toxicity and allergic reactions. Because of the danger to human health, these foods are banned in Europe and many other countries, but are widespread in the American food supply and don't require ANY labeling. The genetically modified foods have no health benefits; the only benefits are the economic ones to the food manufacturers.

If you'd like more information, The Institute for Responsible Technology, the most comprehensive source of GMO information is an excellent resource. Their website: http://www.responsibletechnology.org/.

TIP: The following smartphone apps can assist you in purchasing non-GMO foods:

Non-GMO Project Shopping Guide
Healthy Food, Allergens, GMOs & Nutrition Scanner
True Food
ShopNoGMO
GMO Checker
Chemical Maze
ipiit, The Food Ambassador

The Problem with Today's Wheat

What is the problem with today's modern wheat? It's now just a cheap imitation of the original thing. Advancement in food manufacturing has so drastically changed the structure of wheat from it most natural state, it's just not the same as wheat grown just a few decades ago.

When scientists started cross breeding wheat to make it grow faster and resist its natural dangers (weather and pests), they created a cheaper hybrid product that saved time and money. It's also cultivated to be shorter, doesn't get as much sun, and requires less acreage, but produces more grain. While helping to feed a growing population, this hybrid wheat is having a major impact on our health by causing new allergens and intolerances that many human bodies just can't digest properly – and it's less nutritious. I am one of the millions of people who have developed sensitivity to this new wheat and can only consume it in small doses.

TIP: As you consume wheat (and any product that contains wheat), pay attention to how your body responds. If you have bloating, diarrhea, headache, stomach aches, become sluggish or moody 24 to 48 hours after you consume wheat, you could have a sensitivity or intolerance. If you notice severe reactions after you consume wheat products, see a health professional to determine if you need to remove wheat from you diet.

Pesticides in Our Foods

Pesticides are routinely used in the cultivation of produce, but are toxic by their very nature. After all, they are designed to kill living organisms that threaten food crops. With the national push towards eating more fruits and vegetables, a renewed concern regarding pesticides in our foods is heating up.

According to the Environmental Working Group (EWG) advocacy organization, different pesticides have been linked to a variety of health problems, including:

- Brain and nervous system toxicity
- Cancer
- Hormone disruption
- Skin, eye and lung irritation

Being aware of the foods that have the greatest levels of pesticides is important as you focus on health. With the lists below, it's easy to determine how to be safer from pesticides; they reveal which foods you can buy conventional and which you should spend the extra money on to buy organic.

The Dirty Dozen

Spend the extra money on organic produce whenever possible:

1. Apples
2. Strawberries
3. Grapes
4. Celery
5. Peaches
6. Spinach
7. Sweet Bell Peppers
8. Nectarines- imported
9. Cucumbers
10. Potatoes

11. Cherry Tomatoes
12. Hot Peppers

The Clean 15

Least amount of pesticide contamination you can purchase conventional:

1. Sweet Corn
2. Onions
3. Pineapple
4. Avocado
5. Cabbage
6. Sweet Peas - frozen
7. Papaya
8. Mangos
9. Asparagus
10. Eggplant
11. Kiwi
12. Grapefruit
13. Cantaloupe
14. Sweet Potato
15. Mushrooms

TIP: The thicker the skin on a fruit or vegetable, the less important it is to buy organic (like watermelon or bananas).

TIP: Download the EWP's phone app of the Dirty Dozen and Clean 15 for a more convenient shopping experience.

Trans Fats

Trans Fats (or trans fatty acids) are artificial fats that are created from natural vegetable oils that are pumped with hydrogen to make a solid fat. This new solid fat is then used in processed foods to make them taste better and extend their shelf life. Unfortunately, this fat is unhealthy and can wreak havoc in our bodies. According to the American Heart Association, trans fats:

- Raise your bad (LDL) cholesterol levels
- Lower your good (HDL) cholesterol levels
- Increase your risk of developing heart disease and stroke
- Are associated with a higher risk of developing Type-2 diabetes.

For better health and disease prevention, it's best to avoid trans fats. When grocery shopping for processed foods, look at the ingredient list for the words "partially hydrogenated oils" – which is how trans fats are most commonly listed.

TIP: Beware of foods labeled, "No Trans Fats". The FDA allows any food with less than 0.5 grams of trans fat per serving be labeled as "0" grams or carry a "no trans fat" label.

Not Your Grandfather's Milk

Most modern day dairy cows live in indoor pens their entire lives, which now only average about 5 years. Some are fed diets that include waste from bakeries, soy, and grains; food that cows clearly were not designed to eat. Due to the close confinement and improper diet, many cows get diseased and are given antibiotics. These antibiotics get processed in the end product; the beef and dairy we consume. This has been linked to premature puberty in children.

According to Dr. Joseph Mercola, a world renowned food advocate:

> "Cows that are fed grain and raised under substandard conditions will likely produce milk that is unhealthy to drink raw because grains, antibiotics, growth hormones, and filthy living conditions change the pH balance and the natural bacteria present in a cow's gut, which in turn affects the natural bacteria and pathogens present in their milk."

Additionally, with genetic manipulation, modern cows now produce twice the amount of milk of cows from 50 years ago. Their output is watery milk with half the fat of the cows that are fed green grass. Cows from the 1960s would live for 17-25 years, while cows today only have a life expectancy of about 5 years because of the stressful production environment.

To make cows even more productive and increase profits, some are given Bovine Growth Hormones (BGH), a synthetic hormone. Even though the hormone causes birth defects in calves, the dairy farmers would rather medicate those calves and keep the milk production unnaturally high.

Organic dairy farmers who don't use antibiotics or hormones or take their milk through the traditional pasteurization or homogenized process are not allowed to sell this raw milk for human consumption. Many raw milk advocates will purchase milk from local farmers labeled 'pet milk'.

TIP: If you consume milk, purchase organic milk which doesn't contain hormones or antibiotics.

3
FOOD AS MEDICINE

"Let Food be thy Medicine and Medicine be thy Food."

Hippocrates

Which Foods Are Medicine?

Food Categories

Foods fall into three categories: Carbohydrates, Proteins and Fats. They each have functions and all provide nutrients to our bodies. Let's do a quick overview:

Carbohydrates:

<u>Complex</u> – These foods take longer to digest and provide steady energy from fiber.

Examples: Fruits, vegetables, whole grains, legumes.

<u>Simple</u> – These foods break down very quickly and provide a spike in energy and then a crash.

Examples: Candy bars, soda, cookies, and processed foods.

Proteins:

Protein helps repair our cells, stabilize blood sugar, and burn calories while increasing the feeling of fullness.

Examples: Beef, pork, chicken, fish, eggs, yogurt, cheese, milk, quinoa, soybeans.

Combined Proteins:
Incomplete proteins (beans, peas, whole grains, vegetables, nuts, and seeds) can be combined within 24 hours to make a complete protein. Example: Brown rice and beans, nuts and quinoa, or vegetables and peas will each make a complete protein.

Fats:
Fats in our diet help regulate hormones, cushion organs, assist in brain development and provide energy.
Examples: Butter, olive oil, coconut oil. Fats can also be derived from nuts, seeds and avocados.

TIP: In the process of getting healthier, you should focus on food in the purest form and steer clear of processed foods.

The Best Foods for Health

Consuming more fruits, vegetables and whole grains have been medically proven to improve chronic conditions as well as increase overall well-being. The fact that we can change our health without popping a pill should be very liberating.

Fruits and vegetables have large amounts of antioxidants, a substance that prevents and delays damage to our cells. Cellular damage, called oxidative stress, rusts our bodies on the inside and is caused by aging, consuming unhealthy foods, and by exposure to the environment (like breathing toxic air). Antioxidants found in fruits and vegetables fight oxidative stress. Essentially, foods can either cause this rust in our bodies, or help prevent it.

Research has shown that fruits and vegetables aid in the prevention of cancer based on the review of thousands of research papers commissioned by the World Cancer Research Fund and the American Institute for Cancer Research which states:

The absolute best 7 foods to prevent most chronic disease are:

Tomatoes – Associated with heart health because of the rich amounts of lycopene which studies show lowers a person's risk of cancer. In addition, tomatoes lower LDL cholesterol and triglycerides (a blood lipid that helps move fat and blood glucose from the liver).

Garlic – Has been used for thousands of years as a prescribed medication before pharmaceuticals were invented. Garlic has been proven to lower risks of cancer, improve heart health and reduce high blood pressure.

Broccoli – Has a lot of fiber and reduces the risk of cancer, reverses some heart disease, and prevents osteoporosis.

Carrots – Have high levels of Beta-carotene that converts into vitamin A during digestion.

Strawberries – Help burn stored fat, boost memory, reduce inflammation, promote eye health and boost immunity. Being rich in vitamin C, strawberries also improve your skin's elasticity and resilience.

Spinach – Protects against cancer and is loaded with vitamins A, K, D, and E. Spinach also lowers the acid in our bodies that increases obesity and drains energy.

Green Tea – Contains the most antioxidants of all teas and decreases cancer tumors. Because green tea is the least processed of all tea varieties, it's rich in antioxidant catechins and helps repair cell damage and lowers blood sugar in diabetics.

TIP: The most nutritional benefits are found in raw broccoli so be sure to not overcook it.

Honorable Mentions

In addition to the seven foods mentioned above, there are several other foods that are shown to help prevent disease:

> **Fish** – Consuming fish lowers blood pressure and reduces inflammation while the oils provide nutrients to the brain. Salmon is especially high in omega-3 fatty acids.

> **Mushrooms** – Increase vitamin D production in the body, improve the immune system, and have anti-inflammatory properties that reduce symptoms from asthma, rheumatoid arthritis, renal failure, and stroke damage.

> **Quinoa (And other Whole Grains)** – Pronounced *keen-wah*; quinoa is high in both fiber and protein. It can lower obesity and help prevent breast cancer, heart disease and Type 2 diabetes.

> **Nuts** – Almonds, Brazil nuts, walnuts, hazelnuts and cashews can reduce the risk of heart disease.

Other Healthy Foods

Additional foods that have been proven to fight chronic disease and promote overall good health:

Blackberries	Flaxseed	Legumes	Lemons	Dark Leafy Greens
Whole Grains	Grapefruit	Oranges	Raspberries	Blueberries
Ginseng	Soybeans	Kale	Bok Choy	Sea Cucumber
Pomegranate	Red Wine	Red Grapes	Cherries	Pineapple
Lavender	Artichokes	Nutmeg	Turmeric	Dark Chocolate
Avocado	Parsley	Beets	Apples	Grape Seed Oil
Winter Squash	Olive Oil	Pumpkin	Licorice	

Grass Fed Beef

If you are making progress to get pesticides and hormones out of your food, go a step further and eat grass fed beef, which is much healthier for you than today's mass-produced supermarket beef. Most cows are fed genetically modified corn because it's cheaper – even though cows were created to eat grass.

Grass fed beef has been found to:

- Be lower in total fat
- Have fewer calories
- Contain more heart-healthy omega-3 fatty acids per serving

TIP: Factory farmed beef is cheaper, but making grass fed beef affordable is easy; just reduce your intake by a few ounces and it's the same cost as traditional beef.

DO-IT- YOURSELF Organic Food

As more and more people are taking their health into their own hands, they are turning to aeroponic gardening. This type of gardening grows plants without soil, in air, or mist. Residential aeroponic gardens are now widely available and can provide you a way to grow your own organic, mineral-rich food.

The Tower Garden brands are very popular. For more information and a photo of an aeroponic garden, visit the Reboot Your Life Books website at:

http://www.rebootyourlifebooks.com/ .

4
IT'S NOT JUST ABOUT THE FOOD

"Those who think they have no time for exercise will sooner or later have to find time for illness."

Edward Stanley

Exercise and Your Health

Most people know that exercise improves health, but don't know specifically why and don't make it a priority. Exercising regularly will help your body function better, will help prevent heart disease and diabetes and is a key component in losing weight. Most importantly, people who exercise regularly live longer.

The 2008 *Physical Activity Guidelines for Americans*, compiled by the Department of Health and Human Services describes the major research findings on the health benefits of physical activity:

- Regular physical activity reduces the risk of many adverse health outcomes.
- Some physical activity is better than none.
- For most health outcomes, additional benefits occur as the amount of physical activity increases through higher intensity, greater frequency, and/or longer duration.

- Most health benefits occur with at least 150 minutes (2 hours and 30 minutes) a week of moderate intensity physical activity, such as brisk walking. Additional benefits occur with more physical activity.
- Both aerobic (endurance) and muscle-strengthening (resistance) physical activity are beneficial.
- Health benefits occur for children and adolescents, young and middle-aged adults, older adults, and those in every studied racial and ethnic group.
- The health benefits of physical activity occur for people with disabilities.
- The benefits of physical activity far outweigh the possibility of adverse outcomes, such as injury.

On the other end of the spectrum, the cost of inactivity is huge; increasing the chances of becoming overweight, obese and developing chronic diseases. The Centers for Disease Control reports:

- Americans who live in the South are less active than those who live in the Midwest, Northeast and West.
- More non-Hispanic white adults (22.8%) meet the 2008 Physical Activity Guidelines for aerobic and muscle-strengthening activity than non-Hispanic black adults (17.3%) and Hispanic adults (14.4%).
- Men (52.1%) are more likely than women (42.6%) to meet the 2008 Physical Activity Guideline for aerobic activity.
- Younger adults are more likely to meet the 2008 Physical Activity Guideline for aerobic activity than older adults.

Although starting an exercise program can be challenging if you don't currently workout, it's necessary for good health.

Tip: If you are busy during the day and evening, choose the early morning as your exercise time. If you have limited funds and aren't able to join a gym, walk, find fitness videos on YouTube, or play with your kids—there are many choices that don't require equipment.

Stress and Your Health

Stress, many times called the Silent Killer, can put you at increased risk of numerous health problems if it's not managed properly. The statistics related to stress are staggering:

- 43% of all adults suffer adverse health effects from stress.
- 75% to 90% of all doctor's office visits are for stress-related ailments and complaints.
- The Occupational Safety and Health Administration (OSHA) declared stress a hazard of the workplace.
- Stress now costs American industry more than $300 billion annually.
- Lifetime emotional disorders have increased more than 50%, in large part due to chronic, untreated stress reactions.

According to the Mayo Clinic, the following are very common effects of stress:

On Your Body

Headache

Muscle tension or pain

Chest pain

Fatigue

Change in sex drive

Upset stomach

Sleep problems

On Your Mood

Anxiety

Restlessness

Lack of motivation or focus

Irritability or anger

Sadness or depression

On Your Behavior

Overeating or under eating

Angry outbursts

Drug or alcohol abuse

Tobacco use

Social withdrawal

Often we are not able to remove the main cause of the stress, but finding ways to manage it or limit it can be beneficial to your long term health. Getting a massage, foot reflexology, taking a yoga class, meditating, playing with a baby, or listening to classical music are all activities that will help you to de-stress. Even simple things like going for a walk or taking deep breaths can relieve stress or calm you down in stressful situations.

Leaving stress unmanaged can lead to:

Anxiety	Skin conditions
Asthma	High blood pressure
Arthritis	Heart disease
Diabetes	Sleep problems
Depression	Weight gain
Digestive problems	Memory and concentration impairment

Also, too much stress over a long period of time can lead to many riskier health complications such as strokes and heart attacks. There are many natural supplements that can assist with managing stress, but eliminating the source of your stress is the best scenario, even if it means a drastic life change. This will treat the cause, not the symptom. If you are experiencing any of the symptoms above that aren't alleviated by relaxation methods or other attempts, you should seek medical attention to make sure you aren't doing permanent damage to your body.

TIP: An occasional glass of red wine has proven health benefits, but do not manage stress this way.

Allergens

It's estimated that 1 in 5 Americans have some type of allergy; your body's reaction to substances it believes are harming your body. These substances or allergens can be food, grass, dust, pollen, chemicals, medicine, airborne particles, insect bites or animal hair.

The most common reactions to allergens are sneezing, runny noses, migraine headaches, sore muscles and joints; but in severe cases, death is a risk. In addition to physical reactions, there are behavioral reactions to allergens as well including: crying fatigue, hyperactivity, irritability, sleep disorders, anxiety, and crankiness.

If you have an allergy or intolerance to food and you continue to consume that food, you are doing damage to your body. Severe allergies to gluten found in wheat, barley, and rye causes Celiac disease that can damage your digestive system to the point where the nutrients from foods consumed can't be absorbed. Although there is no cure for Celiac disease, completely removing gluten will clear up the symptoms. If a person with asthma continues to consume dairy, it can lead to more severe asthma attacks that will continue to weaken the respiratory system. We'll learn later that today's dairy causes more mucus to build up in the body so, if you have respiratory problems, do your best to avoid dairy.

Some people can go a lifetime and never have allergies and others are born with them or develop them later in life. Although I've always had an allergy to shellfish, I developed an additional allergy to milk later in life.

The best way to determine if you have allergies or low grade intolerances is to get an allergy test. There are simple online tests for under $100, but the most comprehensive testing has to be done locally by a health professional either with a blood or skin test.

If you can't afford or don't want to take an allergy test, an elimination diet is an easy way to determine if you have an allergy or intolerance to most common foods. This process takes several weeks where you remove the most commonly known allergic foods and slowly add them back, one by one and measure your body's reactions.

The Plan by Lyn-Genet Recitas is an excellent book that walks you through a sophisticated elimination diet. There are also simpler plans online. An elimination diet may not work to identify low grade intolerances so it may be best to move forward with the formal allergy test.

Most Common Food Allergens

Berries	Buckwheat	Chocolate
Cinnamon	Citrus Fruits	Coconut
Dairy Products	Egg Whites	Mustard
Nuts	Peanut Butter	Peas
Pork	Shellfish	Soy
Tomatoes	Wheat	Yeast

For a full list of common foods allergens, visit the Reboot Your Life Books website: http://www.rebootyourlifebooks.com/ .

Since I have full-blown allergies to cow's milk and shellfish, I completely stay away from those foods. With only intolerance to gluten that was developed later in life, I can occasionally consume wheat products, but try to keep it to whole grains.

Regarding milk by-products, I avoid cheese most of the time, but I do still like ice cream. If I consume ice cream, I choose a premium brand, and just eat it in small doses on rare occasions.

If you discover you have intolerance, but still enjoy that food, buy the best quality of that item you can afford but limit consumption to small amounts and rare occasions.

TIP: Always listen to your body, even if the food that seems to be bothering you doesn't show up on an allergy test. For instance, if you know tomatoes cause you problems, avoid them when possible.

Water and Your Health

As most people already know, our bodies can't function properly without water and the lack of water can lead to dehydration and other problems. Our bodies are made up of mostly water and our liver is 96% water.

Drinking water in the proper amounts:

- Increases your brain functions
- Increases your muscle mass
- Flushes toxins
- Helps eliminate fatigue
- Suppresses your appetite which supports weight loss
- Hydrates your skin

Not drinking enough water:

- Damages the kidneys
- Causes stomach pain
- Causes heartburn
- Causes joint pain
- Causes headaches and migraines

Most experts recommend at least 64 ounces (8 one cup servings) of water per day. If you want to lose weight, you should drink a volume of water that is half your body weight in ounces. For instance, if you weigh 150 pounds; you would drink 75 ounces which comes out to a little more than 9 glasses a day. Make sure you consume most of the water outside of your meal time so you won't slow the digestive process.

TIP: To add variety to your daily water intake, infuse with lemon or fruit.

Sleep and Your Health

The National Sleep Foundation cites that 63% of Americans don't get the 8 hours of sleep recommended for good health.

The following conditions have been linked to long term poor sleeping habits: obesity, diabetes, high blood pressure, hypertension, alcohol dependency, depression, and shortened life expectancy. Getting less than 8 hours of sleep a night can weaken your immune system, cause the metabolic process to function improperly, and impair cognitive function.

In order for a person to be healthy, the body needs the appropriate amount of sleep to repair cells, restore energy, balance the appetite, and regulate hormones and other bodily functions.

If a person has interrupted breathing during sleep, they suffer sleep apnea which can lead to serious health issues such as stroke, heart failure and high blood pressure. If you or someone you know has sleep apnea, it is a serious condition that should be treated by a professional.

Although there is always considerable focus on lack of sleep and health risks, over-sleeping is also a health concern. A person that consistently sleeps more than 9 hours a day may have an underlying medical issue that needs attention.

Many people pride themselves on only needing 4 or 5 hours sleep per night. Just because an individual can function on less sleep does not mean they are performing at their best and they certainly aren't able to obtain optimal health on little sleep.

TIP: Limit your digital interactions at least a half hour before bedtime to allow your brain activity to wind down.

Good Dental Health

Practicing good dental health can directly add years to your life. Studies have proven that bacteria can grow in an unhealthy mouth which could lead to respiratory illness, heart disease and diabetes. Be sure to brush your teeth twice a day and floss at least once per day.

Watching the Toilet

A simple way to measure your health at a high level is to become a toilet watcher. Your urine and bowel movement can tell you some basics about your eating habits. The color, smell and shape can give you clues as to how you can improve your eliminations.

Urine

The average adult's urine will total between 5 and 8 cups every 24 hours depending on how much liquid a person consumes. The color of your urine can help indicate if you need more water in your diet.

Urine Colors:

Transparent – Your intake of water is very high, make sure you aren't drinking too much.

Pale Straw Colored – You are drinking the proper amount of water.

Transparent Yellow – This is normal.

Dark Yellow – You should increase your water intake.

Amber or Honey – Your body needs additional water.

Syrupy color – Could be severe dehydration or possible liver disease.

If your urine is cloudy or has an extremely strong order, you should seek out a medical professional to diagnose.

Bowel Movement

Bowel movements should be easy to pass and you should not be straining. Let's take a look at the following from Mercola.com which breaks down healthy vs. unhealthy stools:

Healthy Stool

Medium to light brown.

Smooth and soft, formed into one long shape and not a bunch of pieces.

About one to two inches in diameter and up to 18 inches long.

S-shaped, which comes from the shape of your lower intestine.

Quiet and gentle dive into the water...it should fall into the bowl with the slightest little "whoosh" sound – not a loud, wet cannonball splash that leaves your tush in need of a shower.

Natural smell, not repulsive. (I'm not saying it will smell good!)

Uniform texture.

Sinks slowly.

Unhealthy Stool

Stool that is hard to pass, painful, or requires straining.

Hard lumps and pieces, or mushy and watery, or even pasty and difficult to clean off.

Narrow, pencil-like or ribbon-like stools: can indicate a bowel obstruction or tumor – or worst case, colon cancer; narrow stools on an infrequent basis are not so concerning, but if they persist, definitely warrant a call to your physician.

Black, tarry stools or bright red stools may indicate bleeding in the GI tract; black stools can also come from certain medications, supplements or consuming black licorice; if you have black, tarry stools, it's best to be evaluated by your healthcare provider.

White, pale or gray stools may indicate a lack of bile, which may suggest a serious problem (hepatitis, cirrhosis, pancreatic disorders, or possibly a blocked bile duct), so this warrants a call to your physician; antacids may also produce white stool.

Yellow stools may indicate giardia infection, a gallbladder problem, or a condition known as Gilbert's syndrome – if you see this, call your doctor.

Presence of undigested food (more of a concern if accompanied by diarrhea, weight loss, or other changes in bowel habits).

Floaters or splashers.

Increased mucus in stool: This can be associated with inflammatory bowel disease like Crohn's disease, or ulcerative colitis, or even colon cancer, especially if accompanied by blood or abdominal pain.

For a graphical representation of bowel types, the Bristol Stool Chart can be found on multiple sites on the Internet.

TIP: Check the toilet several times a week to determine if your eliminations are normal.

Environmental Concerns

The environment can play a huge role in your health and everything around you affects your body. There are good elements in the environment, such as the sun, water, and air; and bad elements such as chemicals, pollution, and even noise. Even too much sun can be a hazard.

Taking charge of your health in the environmental area will also allow you to play a role in cleaning up the earth. Being mindful and aware of the environmental hazards can help turn your health in a more positive direction.

Cosmetics and Your Health

I've included this section to make you aware of some of the hidden dangers in the cosmetics that you use every day. There are over 10,000 chemical ingredients in our personal care products (shampoo, conditioners, moisturizers, deodorants, foundations and mascara).

The important thing to note is that some of these chemicals are known or suspected carcinogens; a substance that can cause cancer. Carcinogens are also toxic to the reproductive system and negatively affect the endocrine system. Most chemicals included in our personal care products are at low levels, but if you or members of your family are allergic to any of them, it could be problematic. There are many lines of natural products you can explore if you decide to remove chemicals from your beauty routine.

TIP: If you have a concern about chemicals, or if you or your family uses a lot of personal care items, consider at least switching to natural deodorants and soaps.

Air Quality

Indoor Air Quality

Since we spend most of our time indoors, the air quality as it relates to our health is very important. The American Lung Association says, "Poor indoor air quality can cause or contribute to the development of infections, lung cancer, and chronic lung diseases such as asthma. In addition, it can cause headaches, dry eyes, nasal congestion, nausea and fatigue. People who already have lung disease are at greater risk."

For your health and safety, the Environmental Protection Agency's (EPA) chart below shows the most common indoor pollutants and their effects:

Indoor Air Quality Chart

Pollutant	Sources	Health Effects
Carbon Monoxide (CO)	Furnaces, vehicle exhaust, tobacco smoke, and other combustion processes	Causes angina, impaired vision, and reduced brain function; High concentrations can be fatal.
Carbon Dioxide (CO2)	Human respiration and all combustion processes	Only at high levels, (>1.5% of air or 15,000 ppm), loss of mental acuity noted.
Ozone (O3)	Copy areas and other electrical equipment; Outside air	Decrease in lung function; Aggravation of asthma, chest pain, and inflammation of lung tissue.
Mercury	Medical equipment, electrical switches, some light bulbs, thermostats, and batteries	Cough, chest pain, nausea, diarrhea, long-term weight loss, irritability, and memory loss.
Pesticides	Used in food preparation areas, on indoor plants, wood and other products; Can be tracked in from outside	Depends on active and inert ingredients in the pesticide and the dose received.

Pollutant	Sources	Health Effects
Formaldehyde	Volatilization from building furnishings, certain types of plywood, glues, adhesives, and tobacco smoke	Causes burning in eyes; Irritates mucous membranes and respiratory tract; Probable human carcinogen.
Asbestos	Deteriorating, damaged, or disturbed insulation, fireproofing, acoustical material, and tiles	Causes asbestosis (lung disease), lung, chest, and abdominal cancer; Known human carcinogen.
Volatile Organic Compounds (VOCs)	Paints, cleaners, copiers, tobacco smoke, insecticides, personal care products, and combustion vapors	Some lead to nausea, dizziness, eye, respiratory, and mucous membrane irritation; Some linked to cancer.
Environmental Tobacco Smoke	Tobacco combustion: cigarettes, cigars, pipes	Known human carcinogen; Aggravates asthma.
Nitrogen Oxides	Combustion processes	Eye, respiratory, and mucous membrane irritation; Exacerbates asthma, bronchitis, and emphysema.
Dust	Multiple sources, including soil, fleecy material, pollen, combustion processes, and renovations	Particles may contain lead, pesticide residues, toxic materials, irritants, and/or carcinogens.
Lead	Lead-based paint, drinking water, food, and contaminated soil or air	Damage to brain, kidneys, nervous system, and red blood cells; Children are especially susceptible.
Allergens and Pathogens	Areas of high humidity or significant amounts of moisture; Entrance growth of biological material	Several diseases such as tuberculosis, measles, infections, influenza, Legionnaires disease transmitted by air; Molds and pollen contribute to allergies.

Pollutant	Sources	Health Effects
Radon	Naturally occurring radioactive gas found in earth-ground buildings, well-water, and some materials	Known lung carcinogen.
Polychlorinated Biphenyls	Transformers, capacitors, circuit boards, oils, and other electrical devices	Acute effects unknown; Chronic effects include respiratory, dermal, gastro-intestinal, and reproductive problems. Probable human carcinogen

Outdoor Air Quality Index

The purpose of the Air Quality Index (AQI) is to help you understand what local air quality means to your health. To make it easier to understand, the EPA has divided the AQI into six categories:

Air Quality Index (AQI) Values	Levels of Health Concern	Colors/Meaning
When the AQI is in this range:	*..air quality conditions are:*	*...as symbolized by this color:*
0-50	Good	**Green -** Air quality is considered satisfactory, and air pollution poses little or no risk.
51-100	Moderate	**Yellow -** Air quality is acceptable; however, for some pollutants there may be a moderate health concern for a very small number of people who are unusually sensitive to air pollution.
101-150	Unhealthy for Sensitive Groups	**Orange -** Members of sensitive groups may experience health effects. The general public is not likely to be affected.
151 to 200	Unhealthy	**Red -** Everyone may begin to experience health effects; members of sensitive groups may experience more serious health effects.
201 to 300	Very Unhealthy	**Purple -** Health warnings of emergency conditions. The entire population is more likely to be affected.
301 to 500	Hazardous	**Maroon -** Health alert: everyone may experience more serious health effects

You can find the daily AQI for your city at: http://www.airnow.gov/ .

Household Cleaning Products

Chemicals used in cleaning products are harsh and can cause or aggravate respiratory issues including asthma. Many of the ingredients are carcinogenic or contain preservatives that release low levels of formaldehyde, which can cause cancer.

Whenever I interviewed a new cleaning service, I would ask what type of products they used. I wanted to make sure my house was going to smell fresh after they left. One service told me that they were a natural company and they primarily used vinegar, baking soda and water. I was like, "WHAT??"

The owner informed me that that was the best and most natural way to clean and that I would not be disappointed. I did some research and found out that white distilled vinegar can kill most mold, germs and bacteria and can be used instead of harsh chemicals. I agreed to give the natural service a try and I was pleasantly surprised when the crew left my house, it did smell clean and fresh.

TIP: For routine everyday cleaning, switch to natural cleaning products or homemade ones.

Our Health and Politics

Politics play a huge role in the food industry today and greatly impact the quality of our foods and how they are marketed. Although labeling is required for packaged foods, sometimes it can be quite hard to determine if a food is healthy or harmful. As we've mentioned previously, manufacturers that genetically modify food do not have to disclose that fact. Although consumers are starting to fight back, the food and pesticide manufacturers spent over $70 million to defeat the ballots in California and Washington that would have required GMO labeling.

Consumers are demanding change and are focusing on specific manufacturers. In 2012, there was a huge backlash against General

Mills when it was revealed they donated over a million dollars to fight the anti-GMO labeling laws. General Mills conceded, and is now manufacturing the original Cheerios with all non-GMO products.

Although there is some movement in the right direction, Americans are late to the game; European consumers began rejecting GMO products back in 1999 after scientific research determined consumption of those products was not safe in rats tested. Once the results went public, the outcry was fast and change was swift; European food manufacturers quickly removed GMO ingredients from their products.

Politics is at work in all aspects of the food industry including our schools where unhealthy food continues to be served. Rodale press reports:

> In 2012, The U.S. Department of Agriculture proposed new nutrition standards for meals served in school lunch programs. These specified the numbers and sizes of food servings necessary to meet children's nutritional needs and promote health, but prevent obesity.
>
> Lobbyists for school pizza makers went to work. Bingo! The Senate inserted an amendment to the agriculture spending act, resulting in a dab of tomato paste on pizza counting as a vegetable in school lunches.

If you have children in school, it is in your best interest to find out what type of food is being served so you can decide if you need to pack a healthier lunch.

TIP: If you would like to get involved in the fight to change laws that affect our food supply, visit the Reboot Your Life Books website for a list of grassroots organizations:

http://www.rebootyourlifebooks.com/

Although we can't look to our politicians for direction on our personal health quest, we must be aware of platforms and major laws that may affect us, especially as we learn more about how our processed food is getting less and less nutritious. In the next chapter, we'll learn how we can be less reliant on packaged food and move to more natural foods.

I encourage you to stay informed on what the major political parties have to say about health and healthcare. Below, you'll find the political platform of America's two largest political parties.

Political Platforms on Health - National Democratic Party

http://www.democrats.org/issues/health_care

In March 2010, President Obama fulfilled a promise that Democrats have pursued for nearly a century: making health care available to all Americans. Despite unanimous opposition from Republicans, Democrats were finally able to pass comprehensive health reform into law.

By 2014, health reform will eliminate all discrimination for pre-existing conditions, start the process of expanding health insurance coverage for an additional 32 million Americans, and provide the largest middle-class tax cut for health care in history.

The Affordable Care Act has already begun to end the worst insurance company abuses. Since 2010, children with pre-existing conditions can no longer be denied insurance.

The Affordable Care Act also provides tax cuts to small business to help offset the costs of employee coverage, and tax credits to help families pay for insurance. Health reform will also lower costs for families and for businesses and for the federal government, reducing our deficit by more than $1 trillion in the next two decades alone.

And health reform strengthens Medicare by reducing fraud, improving quality of care, and closing the Medicare "donut hole" gap in seniors' prescription drug coverage.

Like Medicare before it, the Affordable Care Act lays a new foundation for our country that will bring additional security and stability to the American people for generations to come.

Political Platforms on Health - Grand Old Party

http://www.gop.com/2012-republican-platform_Renewing/#Item7

We believe that taking care of one's health is an individual responsibility. Chronic diseases, many of them related to lifestyle, drive healthcare costs, accounting for more than 75 percent of the nation's medical spending. To reduce demand, and thereby lower costs, we must foster personal responsibility while increasing preventive services to promote healthy lifestyles. We believe that all Americans should have improved access to affordable, coordinated, quality healthcare, including individuals struggling with mental illness.

Our goal is to encourage the development of a healthcare system that provides higher quality care at a lower cost to all Americans while protecting the patient-physician relationship based on mutual trust, informed consent, and privileged patient confidentiality. We seek to increase healthcare choice and options, contain costs and reduce mandates, simplify the system for patients and providers, restore cuts made to Medicare, and equalize the tax treatment of group and individual health insurance plans. For most Americans, those who are insured now or who seek insurance in the future, our practical, non-intrusive reforms will promote flexibility in State leadership in healthcare reform, promote a free-market based system, and empower consumer choice. All of which will return direction of the nation's healthcare to the people and away from the federal government.

To return the States to their proper role of regulating local insurance markets and caring for the needy, we propose to block grant Medicaid and other payments to the States; limit federal requirements on both private insurance and Medicaid; assist all patients, including those with pre-existing conditions, through reinsurance and risk adjustment; and promote non-litigation alternatives for dispute resolution. We call on State officials to carefully consider the increased costs of medical mandates, imposed under their laws, which may price many low-income families out of the insurance market. We call on the government to permanently ban all federal funding and subsidies for abortion and healthcare plans that include abortion coverage.

To achieve a free market in healthcare and ensure competition, we will promote price transparency so that consumers will know the actual cost of treatments before they undergo them. When patients are aware of costs, they are less likely to over-utilize services. We support legislation to cap non-economic damages in medical malpractice lawsuits, thereby relieving conscientious providers of burdens that are not rightly theirs and addressing a serious cause of escalating medical bills. We will empower individuals and small businesses to form purchasing pools in order to expand coverage to the uninsured. Individuals with pre-existing conditions who maintain continuous insurance coverage should be protected from discrimination. We support technology enhancements for medical health records and data systems while affirming patient privacy and ownership of health information.

Ensuring Consumer Choice in Healthcare

Consumer choice is the most powerful factor in healthcare reform. Today's highly mobile work force requires portability of insurance coverage that can go with them from job to job. The need to maintain coverage should not dictate where families have to live and work. Putting the patient at the center of policy decisions will increase choice and reduce costs while ensuring that services provide what Americans actually want. We must end tax discrimination against the individual purchase of insurance and allow consumers to purchase insurance across State lines. While promoting "co-insurance" products and alternatives to "fee for service," government must promote Health Savings Accounts and Health Reimbursement Accounts to be used for insurance premiums and should encourage the private sector to rate competing insurance plans. We will ensure that America's aging population has access to safe and affordable care. Because seniors overwhelmingly desire to age at home, we will make home care a priority in public policy. We will champion the right of individual choice in senior care. We will aggressively implement programs to protect against elder abuse, and we will work to ensure that quality care is provided across the care continuum from home to nursing home to hospice.

5
TAKING IT TO THE NEXT LEVEL

"One should eat to live, not live to eat."

Benjamin Franklin

Lifestyle Options

Once you've gotten in the habit of a lifestyle that has improved your health, there are additional steps you can take to strive for optimal health. What exactly is optimal health? If you asked twenty people, you would probably get twenty different answers.

Reaching optimal health means a body that is stress free, disease free, a body that functions as intended, and a life that is balanced in all areas including spiritual, social, etc. Sounds unrealistic? Balancing everything may be tough, but it is attainable.

There are several lifestyle options you can incorporate to take your health to the next level. We'll explore some of the most popular ones.

Vegetarians / Vegan

Vegetarians range from fish and dairy eaters to stricter practices that only include plant based and processed foods. The various approaches are:

> Vegan – Consumes only plant based foods: fruits vegetables, legumes, grains, seeds and nuts.

Lacto-vegetarian – Consumes plant based foods, diet also includes cheese and dairy products.

Ovo-vegetarian – Consumes plant based foods, diet also includes eggs.

Ovo-lacto vegetarian – Consumes plant based foods; diet also includes both eggs and dairy products.

Semi-vegetarians – Consumes plant based foods; diet also includes chicken and fish, dairy products and eggs.

Pescetarian – Consumes plant based foods, diet also includes seafood.

Flexitarian

A flexitarian is a person who has a mostly vegetarian diet, but does eat meat and dairy on occasion. Flexitarian is derived from the two words, flexible and vegetarian. Studies show that vegetarians eat less and weigh less than meat eaters. In this way of eating, your goal is to add more plant based foods to your diet and you don't have to completely give up eating meat forever. There are several books and Internet articles on this subject if you want to delve deeper.

Gluten-Free

Gluten-free eating removes gluten from your diet. Gluten is naturally occurring in wheat, barley, and many processed foods. According to Dr. William Davis, author of *Wheat Belly*, #1 New York Times Best Seller, today's wheat is toxic, addictive, and leads to obesity.

Raw Food Diet

In this eating approach, you can turn off your oven. Raw food eaters believe that heating food destroys all the natural enzymes and nutrients. The staples of the raw food diet are raw fruits, vegetables, nuts, seeds and sprouted grains. Most of the food is eaten raw, but sometimes it is consumed warmed up to 118 degrees.

Clean Eating

Clean Eating is not a clearly definable methodology, but basically followers attempt to avoid processed foods and focus on homemade and organic foods, eating as close to nature as possible.

Clean eaters forgo products and foods with:
- Additives
- Preservatives
- Sweeteners
- Colors
- GMOs
- Hormones
- Antibiotics
- Pesticides and fertilizers

The basic principles of Clean Eating are:
- Eating whole foods
- Avoiding processed foods
- Eating fresh, local, organic fruits and vegetables
- Eliminating refined sugar
- Eating free range and grass-fed meats and dairy
- Eating five or six small meals throughout the day
- Cooking your own meals
- Eating protein/carbohydrate, or
- Carbohydrate/fat for nutritional balance

TIP: If you are considering one of these methodologies, start slowly by taking one day at a time; you don't have to fully commit all at once.

Seek the Appropriate Help

Anyone interested in taking their health to the next level should not do it alone. Many times, individuals do not seek the appropriate healthcare professional before chronic disease or other health issues set in. There are many health markers that indicate if a person is in the 'pre' stages of an illness, such as pre-hypertension, pre-diabetes, etc.

Early detection and taking the appropriate action can prevent the full-blown disease from setting in. As mentioned before, chronic disease is long term and usually not curable. To increase longevity, it is best to aggressively fight to reverse any warning signs of disease as soon as possible and change your lifestyle.

Check in with Your Doctor

Consulting with your doctor before beginning a major lifestyle change is a very important step that many people overlook. An annual check-up will provide you with a baseline of your health markers and record the changes in your body from year to year. Your doctor may also recommend supplements or specific action items you need to incorporate to address any issues uncovered during your visit. Issues that may seem minor could quickly lead to an irreversible chronic illness and hinder your attempts to get healthier and lose weight.

Other Health Professionals

In addition to medical doctors, there are a variety of professionals who can help you on your journey to better health and now many of these services are covered by health insurance:

Natural Doctors / Integrated Medical Facilities

Natural doctors work to find the root cause of a medical issue as opposed to medicating the symptoms. Many of them practice Chinese medicine, iridology, acupuncture, etc. to address the issue from the inside out. They believe in the mind and body connection and prefer to deal with patients who want to look beyond a pharmaceutical solution.

Nutritionist/Dietician

If you were recently diagnosed with a disease, condition or are pre-disposed to getting a chronic disease, your doctor may have referred you to a nutritionist or dietician. They advise people on what to eat in order to lead a healthy lifestyle or achieve a specific health-related goal.

Health Coaches

A Health Coach is a mentor, adviser and supporter who helps you reach your overall wellness goals including weight management, sleep management, increased energy levels and other health improvements. A Health Coach goes beyond what a nutritionist or a dietitian can do; he or she will literally hold your hand and walk you through the process of making a healthy lifestyle change. They can assist you with behavioral choices, typically from a holistic point of view, including mind, body and soul.

A Health Coach is a guide and mentor who empowers clients to take responsibility for his or her own health and supports them to implement and sustain lifestyle and behavior changes that will contribute to the achievement of their personal wellness goals.

Acupuncture

The practice of acupuncture goes back thousands of years and is used for a wide variety of health issues, especially pain management. The technique involves thin solid, metallic needles that penetrate the skin and are manipulated by the practitioner or by electrical stimulation.

Chiropractic Care

Chiropractic care is an alternative form of medicine which not only diagnoses conditions, but also treats the conditions. The practitioner manipulates the spine and joints to align the skeletal system.

Chiropractic care is a very effective method for pain management and lower back issues.

TIP: If you are experiencing a health concern that you've ignored, especially a recurring condition, you should seek the proper attention and take the appropriate steps as directed by your doctor or health care professional.

After you've seen your doctor, it's time to put everything together and set your goals for your health improvement journey. In the following chapter, you'll learn how to set realistic goals and make sure you have the proper support to get started with your new changes.

6
PUTTING IT ALL TOGETHER

**"Whether you think you can, or you think you can't –
you're right."**

Henry Ford

Have the Confidence and Right Attitude

Anytime you embark on a new or unfamiliar adventure, there may be a small crisis of confidence. Don't let fear or any other negative thoughts stop you before you start. Believe that you can make these changes for your health and your family's health. Jot down all the reasons why you want and need to make the changes.

If you are a person of faith, pray daily regarding your health goals and expect that you are going to reach them. Find scriptures or affirmations and review them each morning to give yourself a mental boost.

If you are a parent, one of the greatest gifts you can give your children is to teach them how to be healthy and take care of themselves in the best way possible. If you are a caregiver, you can provide better and healthier options and even improve their lives.

Set Realistic, SMART Goals

No matter what type of health goals you are setting, making them realistic is the key to helping you reach them.

The best goal-setting advice I've found is the SMART method:

> S-Specific
> M-Measurable
> A-Attainable
> R-Relevant
> T-Time Sensitive

Committing to exercise three days a week at the gym when you don't exercise at all is not very attainable. If you currently don't exercise at all, a SMART goal around exercise would be to start working out at home for 15 minutes, two times a week for a month before committing to going to the gym multiple times per week.

The goal above meets all the criteria of a SMART goal because each component is met:

Specific – Begin exercising.
Measurable – Do a work out at home, for 15 minutes, two times per week for one month.
Attainable - Most anyone can find 15 minutes, twice per week to do some form of exercise. Choosing what type of exercise a person would do will really make this goal attainable.
Relevant- Exercise is a huge component of changing your overall health.
Time Sensitive - This goal has a one month timeframe so it doesn't extend too far.

Once the initial month is up, you'll have created an exercise habit that will be easier to transfer to the gym and when obstacles come up, they will be less likely to derail you.

TIP: When setting SMART goals for your food choices, don't try to completely eliminate processed foods immediately if they make up a large part of your current diet. Try replacing one serving of processed food with a healthier choice once per day for a week.

Having the Proper Support

Making changes to your lifestyle to improve your health will take time and adjustments. Because there are so many components these changes should be done over time. Having the proper support will be a key to your success.

If you are married or have a family, get them on board to make sure you stay focused and on track. If you are unable to get support from your immediate family, reach out to friends or create your own support group. With today's technology, your support group doesn't even need to be local. You can easily create a secret group on Facebook or use a smartphone app like MyFitnessPal to connect with your support team. In addition to your support team, get one or two accountability partners that you 'report' in to several times per week.

Charting Your Success

As you are moving towards your health goals, be sure to chart your progress and noticeable improvements. There are several ways you can measure your success.

Health Markers: Results from your doctor's office are a great way to measure your success. If you have made drastic changes in your health, you may want to schedule a 6-month follow-up visit and have you doctor compare your "before and after" results.

Weight Loss: When you change your eating and health habits for the better, you will lose weight. Your rate of weight loss will depend upon how you approach your changes. Weight loss is 80% nutrition and 20% fitness; if you focus first on eating fewer processed foods and more fresh fruits, vegetables and lean proteins you will lose weight at a more rapid pace.

Body Measurements: Use a measuring tape to measure your before and after results As you change your lifestyle to a healthier one, you'll begin to notice your clothes are looser.

Energy Level: Once processed foods are flushed out of your system, you will likely feel your energy increase. If your body is free of unhealthy foods, your organs will be able to focus on their normal functions instead of trying to process chemicals.

Sleep: As your body becomes healthier it will begin to self-regulate, and one area that changed for me was my sleep patterns. After reducing stress, my sleep improved greatly. Signs of improved health can show up in your sleep in the form of deeper sleep, falling asleep easier and waking up easier.

Skin: Our skin improves from the inside out and those improvements can show up in a matter of days with a change to a healthier diet. Our entire body, including the skin, is constantly under construction, and uses all the nutrients and vitamins from our food to rebuild and repair its cells.

Hair: Dermatologist Dr. Amy McMichael explains, "Healthy hair is hair that's growing appropriately out of every follicle, not easily broken, and connected to a healthy scalp.... its hair that's as long and full as you'd like it to be. Since hair is mostly protein, getting the proper amount of lean protein is important to healthy hair. As you switch to leaner, less fatty meats, look for stronger and shinier hair."

Gums: If you have bleeding gums, improving your diet can help; sugar and refined carbohydrates feeds plaque.

Nails: Your fingernails are also primarily protein so healthier eating habits can also improve your nails.

A companion to this book is the *Reboot Your Life: The Easy Start Guide to Making Health Changes Stick Journal* which you can use to chart your success. You can order the book from Amazon or the Reboot Your Life Books website: http://www.rebootyourlifebooks.com/

TIP: After you've established healthier habits and noticed your body's changes, reward yourself: take an hour off to take a bubble bath, read a book or magazine.

Now that you've learned about goal setting, the next chapter will lay out the flexible program to reboot your life and make healthy changes stick. You'll find out just how easy it is to incorporate healthy changes into your life.

7

7 EASY WAYS TO REBOOT YOUR LIFE

"A man too busy to take care of his health is like a mechanic too busy to take care of his tools."

Spanish Proverb

YOU HAVE THE POWER

The power is in your hands to make your lifestyle change! I'll show you how seven easy choices will make the changes almost seamless.

Because there are so many components to consider when making a major change, I've made a list of actions items, which I call Health Boosters that will make it easy to make that change.

The Health Boosters are divided into seven categories, which I'll call The 7 Pillars of Health. The seven pillars are:

1. General Health

2. Food Related

3. On The Go

4. Meals

5. Exercise

6. Spirituality

7. The Next Level

The beauty is you get to choose the Health Boosters you want to work on; what's best for you and your family for that week. These choices will allow you the flexibility to make healthy choices based on your circumstances, not a strict set of rules.

Let's Get Started

Step One: On the next several pages, you'll find 98 Health Boosters in matrix form, categorized by each health pillar. First, read all the way through the list of Health Boosters. Once you've read through the entire matrix of Health Boosters, decide on one item from each health pillar that you would like to work on for the week. Think about your upcoming week; will you have to face a hurdle this week that might affect your ability to focus on your health? Is it a light week where you'll have an opportunity to select more challenging Health Boosters? You decide. Take a look at the sample on page 64. Record on a blank form starting on page 69 and track your progress for the week.

Health Boosters

General Health	Food Related	On The Go	Meals	Exercise	Spirituality	The Next Level
1) Drink at least 8 glasses of water per day	2) Remove sodas and sweet drinks	3) Order a wine spritzer instead of a mixed drink	4) Eat meat only once per day this week	5) Exercise one day this week (if you don't currently exercise)	6) Keep a Positive Mental Attitude	7) Drink the amount of water equal to ½ your body weight in oz. every day (150lb person would drink 75 oz.)
8) Do not add additional salt to your food	9) Eat an apple a day this week	10) When eating out, order a salad with balsamic dressing	11) Have one meatless meal this week	12) Play with your kids one day this week	13) Keep a food journal each day this week	14) Eliminate all known allergens
15) Take the appropriate supplement each day	16) Remove all white food from your diet one day this week	17) Prepare small bag of healthy foods for on-the-go snacking (carrots, grapes, sliced cucumber)	18) Replace 3 meals per week with a protein shake	19) Do 25 jumping jacks each day this week	20) Pray or Meditate daily about your health	21) Remove dairy from your diet
22) Eliminate artificial sugars	23) Replace sodas with plain seltzer water	24) Keep low calorie snacks readily available	25) Replace one meal per day with a bean soup	26) Wear an activity tracker (Fitbit, etc.) and track your progress	27) Give someone a hug every day this week	28) Remove gluten and wheat from your diet

Health Boosters

General Health	Food Related	On The Go	Meals	Exercise	Spirituality	The Next Level
29) Do not 'clean your plate' if you are already full	30) Eat grass fed beef	31) When eating out, split a meal with others	32) Have fish as the main protein for one meal	33) When running errands, park as far away as possible from the entrance	34) Take a stress relieving walk 2x this week	35) Remove corn from your diet
36) Drink a cup of green tea daily	37) Eat broccoli, cabbage, cauliflower or spinach 2x this week	38) When eating out, order grilled, steamed or sautéed entrees	39) Cook two slow cooker meals	40) Stretch before getting out of bed 3x this week	41) Take 30 minutes to decompress outside at the beach, mountains or a park	42) Replace peanut butter with almond butter
43) Get 8 hours of sleep	44) Eat kale 1x this week	45) When eating out, do not eat fast food	46) Eliminate your nightly snack	47) Exercise 3x this week	48) Take a yoga class once this week	49) Use hummus instead of mayonnaise
50) Eat breakfast every day	51) Eat only berries as a snack	52) Order a vegetable plate when eating out	53) Eat meals on a smaller plate	54) Do strength training 2x this week	55) Stop eating when you are full	56) Eat before 7pm each day
57) Floss your teeth at least 1x per day	58) Do not eat any sweets (cakes, candy, cookies, etc.)	59) When eating out, order water instead of a soda or tea	60) Plan your lunch and dinner this week	61) Work with a personal trainer	62) Tell someone you love them each day	63) Switch to almond or rice milk

Health Boosters

General Health	Food Related	On The Go	Meals	Exercise	Spirituality	The Next Level
64) Eliminate all alcohol	65) Remove carbonated drinks	66) When eating out, order fish instead of beef or chicken	67) Add quinoa to one meal	68) Take an exercise class with your spouse	69) Choose a scripture or affirmation and repeat 3x each morning	70) Eat intuitively, only when you are truly hungry
71) Eat more slowly and put your fork down between bites	72) Do not eat any fried foods	73) When eating out, leave the sauce or mayonnaise off your meal	74) Make a meal plan for the week	75) Plan a family outdoor event	76) Take three deep breaths 3x a day	77) Don't eat foods with ingredients you can't pronounce
78) Weigh yourself once per week	79) Eat free range chicken	80) When eating out, choose a leaner cut of beef	81) Eat half of your normal portion this week	82) Learn a new sport	83) Meditate for 10 minutes each day	84) Eat only organic meat
85) Educate yourself – read one health article this week	86) Eat only cage-free eggs	87) When eating out, order marinara sauce instead of creamier sauces	88) Replace vegetable oils with coconut oil	89) Work out 4x this week	90) Help someone less fortunate one day this week	91) Take a whole food supplement daily
92) Switch your normal salad dressing to balsamic vinegar and oil	93) Replace fruit juice with a piece of actual fruit	94) When eating out, do not eat from the bread bowl	95) Eat chemical free for one day this week	96) Do 20 crunches at least 5 days this week	97) Listen to classical music 3x this week	98) Don't eat GMO foods

SAMPLE MATRIX

Health Pillars	#	Health Booster	MON	TUE	WED	THU	FRI	SAT	SUN
General Health	36	Drink a cup of green tea daily							
Food Related	72	Do not eat any fried foods this week							
On the Go	31	When eating out, split a meal with others							
Meals	67	Add quinoa to one meal this week							
Exercise	19	Do 25 jumping jacks per day this week							
Spiritual	69	Choose a scripture or affirmations repeat 3x a day							
The Next Level	91	Take a whole food supplement daily							

Once you've completed one week, select another seven items to focus on for the next week. For week two, three, and four, choose another seven Health Boosters. For week five, determine which seven Health Boosters are most comfortable for your lifestyle and make the change for two straight months instead of one week.

The blank charts will change to reflect Month and Week (M1 – W1, etc.) to track your progress. Once you've gotten through two months of the same seven Health Boosters, try another seven Health Boosters and make them more challenging. Focusing on seven Health Boosters for two months will allow you to make the change permanent.

If you want a more detailed and a comprehensive health program, the Reboot Your Life System is available on the Reboot Your Life Books website: http://www.rebootyourlifebooks.com/

Taking it Slow for Permanent Change

Creating a permanent change takes more than the short 21 days we've been told in the past. According to Dr. Caroline Leaf, Christian neuroscientist, "It takes 21 days to break down a negative toxic pattern and an additional two cycles of 21 days minimum to automatize (make a habit) the new way of thinking."

The three cycles means it will take at least 63 days to make a lasting change.

Although taking it slow won't create the quick and dramatic weight loss that most of us want to see, it will set you up for a healthier lifestyle and make you more aware of your everyday choices, food and exercise which will eventually lead to better health and weight loss.

CONCLUSION
"Knowledge is Power but Action Gets Things Done."

Anonymous

What You've Learned

Now that you know the most important factors that concern your health, you have all the tools to start your journey. The power is in your hands and you have the flexibility to start easy and step it up to more challenging healthy habits when you're ready.

What I hoped to accomplished was to show that nutrition is the key to better health and that average people can get better health. You've learned that you don't have to be an expert on health and can make healthy changes no matter how hectic your lifestyle.

If you're a parent, one of the best gifts you can give your children is the gift of good health. Teaching your kids how to make the best choices for their health at an early age will help prevent disease and will set them up for long and healthy lives.

For most of us, good health is an attainable goal that can be reached by first making easy changes, practicing the habit to make those changes permanent, and then progressing to the next level for optimal health.

Taking Action

Now it's time to take action and start your journey. It's fine to begin slowly; the important thing is that you start to make your change so you can improve your health.

Think about this time next year; how much better will your health be if you begin your changes today? Think about how good you'll feel one year from now after you've consistently put healthier foods in your body. Next year will come whether you take action or not, so go ahead and get started now and Reboot Your Life!

Additional Resources and Support

Reboot Your Life Books Website

A comprehensive resource with everything you need to make lasting changes to live a healthier life. You can find information on all the additional resources listed at:

http://www.rebootyourlifebooks.com/

Personal Health Coach – If you feel that you need the services of a certified health coach, to assist you with your health changes, contact the author through the Reboot Your Life Books website.

Reboot Your Life System – An in-depth program based on the Health Boosters that incorporates recipes, meal planning, and additional information on health and the benefits of good nutrition. See the Reboot Your Life Books website to learn more.

Reboot Your Life Today - The Easy Start Guide to Make Health Changes Stick Journal – A companion guide/food journal that allows you to stay motivated, track your goals and chart your progress in a unique layout for easy recording. Order at www.amazon.com or the Reboot Your Life Books website.

WEEK ONE: Date_____ Weekly Scripture / Affirmation_____

Health Pillars	#	Health Booster	MON	TUE	WED	THU	FRI	SAT	SUN
General Health									
Food Related									
On the Go									
Meals									
Exercise									
Spiritual									
The Next Level									

WEEK TWO: Date_____ Weekly Scripture / Affirmation_____

Health Pillars	#	Health Booster	MON	TUE	WED	THU	FRI	SAT	SUN
General Health									
Food Related									
On the Go									
Meals									
Exercise									
Spiritual									
The Next Level									

WEEK THREE: Date_____ Weekly Scripture / Affirmation_____

Health Pillars	#	Health Booster	MON	TUE	WED	THU	FRI	SAT	SUN
General Health									
Food Related									
On the Go									
Meals									
Exercise									
Spiritual									
The Next Level									

WEEK FOUR: Date_____   Weekly Scripture / Affirmation_____

Health Pillars	#	Health Booster	MON	TUE	WED	THU	FRI	SAT	SUN
General Health									
Food Related									
On the Go									
Meals									
Exercise									
Spiritual									
The Next Level									

M1 -W1: Date_____ Weekly Scripture / Affirmation_____

Health Pillars	#	Health Booster	MON	TUE	WED	THU	FRI	SAT	SUN
General Health									
Food Related									
On the Go									
Meals									
Exercise									
Spiritual									
The Next Level									

M1 –W2: Date_____   Weekly Scripture / Affirmation_____

Health Pillars	#	Health Booster	MON	TUE	WED	THU	FRI	SAT	SUN
General Health									
Food Related									
On the Go									
Meals									
Exercise									
Spiritual									
The Next Level									

M1 –W3: Date_____   Weekly Scripture / Affirmation_____

Health Pillars	#	Health Booster	MON	TUE	WED	THU	FRI	SAT	SUN
General Health									
Food Related									
On the Go									
Meals									
Exercise									
Spiritual									
The Next Level									

M1 –W4: Date_____ Weekly Scripture / Affirmation_____

Health Pillars	#	Health Booster	MON	TUE	WED	THU	FRI	SAT	SUN
General Health									
Food Related									
On the Go									
Meals									
Exercise									
Spiritual									
The Next Level									

M2 -W1: Date_____   Weekly Scripture / Affirmation_____

Health Pillars	#	Health Booster	MON	TUE	WED	THU	FRI	SAT	SUN
General Health									
Food Related									
On the Go									
Meals									
Exercise									
Spiritual									
The Next Level									

M2 –W2: Date_____ Weekly Scripture / Affirmation_____

Health Pillars	#	Health Booster	MON	TUE	WED	THU	FRI	SAT	SUN
General Health									
Food Related									
On the Go									
Meals									
Exercise									
Spiritual									
The Next Level									

M2 –W3: Date_____ Weekly Scripture / Affirmation_____

Health Pillars	#	Health Booster	MON	TUE	WED	THU	FRI	SAT	SUN
General Health									
Food Related									
On the Go									
Meals									
Exercise									
Spiritual									
The Next Level									

M2 –W4: Date_____ Weekly Scripture / Affirmation _____

Health Pillars	#	Health Booster	MON	TUE	WED	THU	FRI	SAT	SUN
General Health									
Food Related									
On the Go									
Meals									
Exercise									
Spiritual									
The Next Level									

M3 -W1: Date_____   Weekly Scripture / Affirmation_____

Health Pillars	#	Health Booster	MON	TUE	WED	THU	FRI	SAT	SUN
General Health									
Food Related									
On the Go									
Meals									
Exercise									
Spiritual									
The Next Level									

M3 –W2: Date_____ Weekly Scripture / Affirmation_____

Health Pillars	#	Health Booster	MON	TUE	WED	THU	FRI	SAT	SUN
General Health									
Food Related									
On the Go									
Meals									
Exercise									
Spiritual									
The Next Level									

M3 –W3: Date_____ Weekly Scripture / Affirmation_____

Health Pillars	#	Health Booster	MON	TUE	WED	THU	FRI	SAT	SUN
General Health									
Food Related									
On the Go									
Meals									
Exercise									
Spiritual									
The Next Level									

M3 –W4: Date_____   Weekly Scripture / Affirmation_____

Health Pillars	#	Health Booster	MON	TUE	WED	THU	FRI	SAT	SUN
General Health									
Food Related									
On the Go									
Meals									
Exercise									
Spiritual									
The Next Level									

WEEK ____ : Date _____ Weekly Scripture / Affirmation _____

Health Pillars	#	Health Booster	MON	TUE	WED	THU	FRI	SAT	SUN
General Health									
Food Related									
On the Go									
Meals									
Exercise									
Spiritual									
The Next Level									

WEEK _____ : Date _____ Weekly Scripture / Affirmation _____

Health Pillars	#	Health Booster	MON	TUE	WED	THU	FRI	SAT	SUN
General Health									
Food Related									
On the Go									
Meals									
Exercise									
Spiritual									
The Next Level									

WEEK _____ ; Date_____ Weekly Scripture / Affirmation_____

Health Pillars	#	Health Booster	MON	TUE	WED	THU	FRI	SAT	SUN
General Health									
Food Related									
On the Go									
Meals									
Exercise									
Spiritual									
The Next Level									

WEEK _____ : Date_____ Weekly Scripture / Affirmation_____

Health Pillars	#	Health Booster	MON	TUE	WED	THU	FRI	SAT	SUN
General Health									
Food Related									
On the Go									
Meals									
Exercise									
Spiritual									
The Next Level									

WEEK ____ : Date _____ Weekly Scripture / Affirmation _____

Health Pillars	#	Health Booster	MON	TUE	WED	THU	FRI	SAT	SUN
General Health									
Food Related									
On the Go									
Meals									
Exercise									
Spiritual									
The Next Level									

WEEK _____ : Date_____ Weekly Scripture / Affirmation_____

Health Pillars	#	Health Booster	MON	TUE	WED	THU	FRI	SAT	SUN
General Health									
Food Related									
On the Go									
Meals									
Exercise									
Spiritual									
The Next Level									

WEEK ____ : Date _____ Weekly Scripture / Affirmation _____

Health Pillars	#	Health Booster	MON	TUE	WED	THU	FRI	SAT	SUN
General Health									
Food Related									
On the Go									
Meals									
Exercise									
Spiritual									
The Next Level									

WEEK _____ : Date _____ Weekly Scripture / Affirmation _____

Health Pillars	#	Health Booster	MON	TUE	WED	THU	FRI	SAT	SUN
General Health									
Food Related									
On the Go									
Meals									
Exercise									
Spiritual									
The Next Level									

WEEK____ : Date_____ Weekly Scripture / Affirmation_____

Health Pillars	#	Health Booster	MON	TUE	WED	THU	FRI	SAT	SUN
General Health									
Food Related									
On the Go									
Meals									
Exercise									
Spiritual									
The Next Level									

NOTES

www.ingramcontent.com/pod-product-compliance
Lightning Source LLC
Chambersburg PA
CBHW060419290526
45791CB00002B/823